Southern Paleo

50 Easy and Delicious Gluten Free Recipes from Down South

Disclaimer
©All Rights Reserved

Contents

Stir-Fried Bacon
Serves 2

Cooking Time

45 minutes

Ingredients

Avocado, 1
Bacon Slices (diced), 8
Black Pepper (freshly grounded)
Sweet Potato (diced), 1 medium
Yellow Onion (diced), ½
Zucchini (diced), 1 medium

Directions
1. Heat a medium skillet over medium-low heat and cook the bacon. Set aside.

2. Take a large sauté pan and heat over medium-high heat. Add onion, sweet potato and 1 tablespoon of bacon fat dripping from the cooked bacon.

3. Cook for about 10-15 minutes while stirring often. Add zucchini and cook.

1. Add bacon and vegetables to the mixture. Season with pepper and avocado. Enjoy!

Omelet Muffins
Serves 4

Cooking Time

40 minutes

Ingredients

Bacon (cooked), 6 strips
Broccoli, ½ cup
Eggs, 12
Pepper
Salt

Directions

1. Preheat the oven to 350°. Take a muffin tin and grease it.

2. Cook the bacon in the oven.

3. Meanwhile, steam the broccoli.

4. After the broccoli is steamed, rinse, drain and chop it into small pieces.

5. Take a large bowl and whisk the eggs, salt and pepper. Add bacon and broccoli and mix well.

6. Put the mixture in the muffin tin and bake for 20-25 minutes.

7. Eat when it is totally cooked and the tops are crisp and brown.

Peppermint Patties
Serves 2-3

Cooking Time

25 minutes

Ingredients

Chocolate chips, 1 cup
Coconut (unsweetened and shredded), 1 cup
Coconut milk, 2 tablespoons
Coconut oil, 2 tablespoons
Honey, ¼ cup
Peppermint extract, ¼ teaspoon

Directions

1. In a food processor, add the shredded coconut and process for 30 seconds.

2. Add remaining ingredients (except the chocolate chips) and process again to form a smooth paste.

3. In 1 ½ inch size rounds, shape the paste to form the patties and place them on a cookie sheet.

4. For 10 minutes, put the sheet in the freezer.

5. Using the microwave or a double broiler, melt the chocolate.

6. Take the patties out of the freezer and add the chocolate.

7. Allow to harden before serving. Enjoy!

Southern Paleo Mushroom and Onions Steak
Serves 4

Cooking Time

15 minutes

Ingredients

Beef (Thin strips or thin cut round sandwich steaks), ½ lb
Extra virgin olive oil. 3 teaspoon
Garlic Powder, to taste
Mushrooms (fresh and sliced), 8 ozs
Pepper (fresh and cracked), to taste
Salt, to taste
Yellow Onions (sliced into rings), ½ large

Directions

1. Season the beef with salt, pepper and garlic. Set aside.

2. Take a large skillet and heat over high heat. add 1 tsp olive oil and half of the beef.

3. Cook 1 minute, turn and cook for 30 seconds. Set aside in a large dish.

4. Repeat process for the remaining beef and add to the dish.

5. Sauté onion in a tsp of olive oil. Season with salt and pepper and cook for about a minute while turning or until they are golden.

6. Bring the heat to medium and add olive oil, mushrooms, salt and pepper. Spray the top of the mushrooms and cook for 1 ½ minute. Turn and cook for another 1 minute.

7. Add to the dish, stir and serve.

Paleo Almond Hot Chocolate
Serves 1

Cooking Time

2-3 minutes

Ingredients

70% Dark Chocolate (melted with 2 tablespoons of hot water), 2 tasting squares
Ground Cinnamon, a dash
Pure Organic Vanilla Extract, ¼ tea spoon
Vanilla Almond milk (warm and unsweetened), 1 cup

Directions

Blend all the ingredients together and serve warm. Enjoy!

Lime and Tequila Chicken
Serves 6

Cooking Time

25 minutes

Ingredients

Chicken breasts (skinless and boneless), 6
Cilantro (fresh and chopped), ½ bunch
Garlic, 5 cloves
Jalapeno (sliced), 1
Limes, 4
Olive oil, ¼ cup
Tequila, 1 cup

Directions

1. Take a food processor or blender, squeeze out the juice of the limes and add salt, olive oil, tequila, garlic, cilantro and jalapeno. Blend well.

2. In a large plastic bag, add the chicken and lime-tequila mixture. Marinate the sealed bag placed in the fridge for about 4-6 hours or overnight if possible.

3. Take out chicken from the bag. Grill over medium-high heat until the chicken is cooked, turning it to cook each side for 4-5 minutes.

Tip: Serve withPico de Gallo sauce for added flavor.

Paleo Roasted Asparagus
Serves 4

Cooking Time

20 minutes

Ingredients

Almonds or pine nuts, ¼ cup
Asparagus spears, 1 ½ pounds (approx. 30 spears)
Garlic salt, ¼ teaspoon
Ghee (melted), 2 tablespoons
Nutmeg, ¼ teaspoon
Olive oil, 1 tablespoon

Directions

1.Preheat the oven to 425°F.

2. Rinse the asparagus and break off the stalks from the ends to about 1-2 inches.

3. Take a large foil-lined baking pan and place the asparagus in a single layer. Roll to coat in drizzled oil.

4. Roast in oven for 10 minutes or until tender-crisp.

5. Add salt, nutmeg, red pepper and butter. Pour mixture over the asparagus and garnish with almonds/pine nuts.

Tasty Paleo Herb Salmon
Serves 4

Cooking Time

20 minutes

Ingredients

Dill (fresh and chopped), 2 tablespoons
Extra virgin olive oil (divided), 6 tablespoons
Leek (sliced), 1
Lemon juice of ½ a lemon
Onion (chopped), 1
Parsley (fresh and chopped), 2 tablespoons
Salmon fillets, 4-5 oz
Salt and pepper to taste
White wine (dry), ½ cup

Directions

1. Wash the fillets and pat dry using paper towels. In a bowl and add the fillets and the wine. Keep cool for about 30 minutes.

2. Preheat the oven to 400°F.

3. In a small bowl, stir in the herbs, salt, lemon juice, salt and pepper and 5 tablespoons of olive oil. Set aside.

4. Carefully arrange the fillets on a shallow ovenproof dish. Make sure to keep a distance of 1-inch between each.

5. Heat a skillet over medium flame. Stir in the onions, leeks and remaining olive oil. Cook for 4 minutes while stirring occasionally. Remove from heat and pour evenly divided portions over the fish to coat each side properly.

6. Place in oven for 10 minutes or until cooked.

7. Serve immediately!

Paleo Strawberry Muffins
Serves 8

Cooking Time

35 minutes

Ingredients

Almond flour, 2 cups
Baking soda, ½ teaspoon
Coconut oil (melted), 1 tablespoon
Eggs, 3
Fresh strawberries (chopped), 1 cup
Ghee (melted), 1 tablespoon
Honey, ¼ cup
Lemon juice, 1 tablespoon
Salt, 1/8 teaspoon
Vanilla extract, 1 teaspoon

Directions

1. Preheat the oven to 325° F.

2. Grease the muffin tins.

3. Take a large and a medium bowl. In the large bowl, combine all dry ingredients and in the medium bowl combine all wet ingredients. Mix the wet ingredients into the dry ones to form a paste.

4. Fold the strawberries in the mixture and using a scoop, pour in the strawberry mixture into the muffin cups. Fill about ¾ of the cup.

5. Bake for about 20-25 minutes or until golden brown.

Paleo Pumpkin Muffins
Serves 4-6

Cooking Time

30 minutes

Ingredients

Almond butter, 1 cup
Almond flour, 1 cup
Baking soda, ½ teaspoon
Cinnamon, ½ teaspoon
Coconut oil, 1/3 cup
Eggs (whisked), 3
Pecans (chopped), ½ cup
Pumpkin (canned), 1 cup
Raw honey, ½ cup
Salt, ¼ teaspoon

Directions

1. Preheat the oven to 350° F.

2. Take a large bowl and mix salt, cinnamon, baking soda and almond flour in it.

3. Mix in the eggs, honey, pumpkin, almond butter and coconut oil.

4. Add chopped pecans to the mixture.

5. Grease muffin tins and pour in the mixture in equal amounts.

6. Bake for about 15-20 minutes.

Grilled Paleo Chicken
Serves 8

Cooking Time

50 minutes

Ingredients

Balsamic vinegar, 1 tablespoon
Black pepper (coarse), ¼ teaspoon
Bone-in Chicken parts, 3 ½ pounds
Chili powder, 1 tablespoon
Cinnamon, 1 tablespoon
Cocoa powder (unsweetened), 1 teaspoon
Olive oil, 3 tablespoons
Organic coconut sugar (Madhava), 1 tablespoon
Salt, ½ teaspoon

For the Lime Butter:

Black pepper (coarse), 1 pinch
Fresh Cilantro (chopped), ¼ cup
Ghee (melted), ½ cup
Lime juice (fresh), 1 tablespoon
Serrano pepper (minced), 1
White onion (minced), 2 tablespoons

Directions

1. Blend in the vinegar, pepper, chili powder, cinnamon, olive oil, coconut sugar, salt and cocoa powder in a small bowl

2. Using a basting brush or a spoon spread the seasoning over the chicken

3. Grill the chicken for 30 minutes or until cooked (for a gas grill use medium heat and for a charcoal grill use indirect heat)

4. In a small bowl, add all the ingredients for the lime butter.

5. Serve the chicken with lime butter topping or as a dip.

Paleo Lamp Chops
Serves 4

Cooking Time

15 minutes

Ingredients

Black pepper (freshly grounded), 1 teaspoon
Extra virgin olive oil (divided), 4 tablespoons
Garlic (minced), 1 clove
Lamb chop (ribs attached), 1 pound
Rosemary (fresh and minced), 3 tablespoons
Salt, 2 teaspoons

Directions

1. Prior to starting, mix the ingredients well and marinate the lamb chops for about 4 hours and get to room temperature about 30 minutes before cooking.

2. In an ovenproof sauté pan, heat up 2 tablespoons of oil over high flame. Add lamb chops to shimmering hot oil and sear each side for 2-3 minutes.

3. Remove from heat, cover and set aside. Allow them to resettle before serving.

If you want them cooked more, you can bake them in the oven for 3-5 minutes at 400 F. Again, allow to rest before serving.

Paleo Chicken Nuggets
Serves 4

Cooking Time

20-25 minutes

Ingredients

Almond flour, 1 cup
Chicken breasts, 2
Eggs, 2
Garlic powder
Mozzarella cheese, ½ cup (or as desired)
Olive oil, ½ cup
Onion powder
Salt and pepper to taste

Directions

1. Heat the oil in a saucepan.

2. Make small bit size pieces of the chicken and set aside.

3. Take a bowl and scramble both eggs in it.

4. Make a mix of onion powder, garlic powder, salt and pepper to season the nuggets

5. Dip each nugget first in the eggs, then in seasoning mix and place it into the saucepan.

6. Cook each side of the nugget for 2-3 minutes or until golden brown.

7. Serve warm and enjoy!

Paleo Almond Crust Pizza
Serves 4

Cooking Time

60 minutes

Ingredients

For Crust:
Almond flour, 3 cups
Butter, 1 stick
Eggs, 6
Garlic powder, 1-2 tablespoons

For Toppings:
Bacon (chopped), 3 slices
Olive oil, 2 teaspoon (for topping)
Pepperoni
Red pepper flakes, 1 tablespoon
Tomato sauce, ½ - 1 cup (optional)
Mozzarella Cheese, 1-2 cups or as desired
Garlic (minced), 3-4 cloves
Mushrooms (sliced and cut), 10-15

Directions

1. Preheat oven to 350° F.

2. Take a large bowl and beat in the 6 eggs.

3. Add in butter, flour and garlic powder. Mix well.

4. Place on a pan, spread well to form a ½ - ¼ layer. Cook the crust in the oven for 10-15 minutes.

5. Meanwhile, sauté the toppings using 2 teaspoons olive oil in a pan.

6. Remove crust from oven. Cook toppings further if needed.

7. Spread sauce over the crust and add toppings.

8. Place in oven for another 25-30 minutes.

Paleo Red Curry Beef
Serves 4-6

Cooking Time

4 hours

Ingredients

Beef (cut into fajita strips), 2-3 pounds
Coconut milk, 1 can
Garlic (minced), 2 cloves
Red curry paste, 3 tablespoons
Red pepper flakes, 1 tablespoon

Directions

1. Take a slow cooker and add in all the ingredients. Stir well.

2. Cover and cook on low heat for 4 hours.

3. Place over potatoes or rice.

4. Serve warm!

Coconut Cream of Broccoli Soup
Serves 2-3

Cooking Time

6-8 hours

Ingredients

Broccoli florets, 5 cups
Celery stalks (diced), 4
Chicken broth, 2 cups
Coconut flour, 3 tablespoons
Coconut milk, 1 can
Coconut oil, 3 tablespoons
Garlic (minced), 3 cloves
Yellow onion (diced), 1 medium
Seasonings as per taste (basil, garlic powder, pepper, red pepper, salt, thyme and onion powder)

Directions

1. Take 1 tablespoon of coconut oil and sauté the celery, garlic and onions.

2. In a slow cooker, pour in the mixture.

3. Heat the remaining coconut oil in the same pot/pan and whisk in the coconut flour being careful not to form lumps.

4. Whisk in the coconut milk and mix well. Add to the slow cooker along with the broth and the spices.

5. Stir in the broccoli and cover.

6. Cook for 6-8 hours and enjoy.

Paleo Tomato Salad
Serves 2

Cooking Time

10 Minutes

Ingredients

Cucumbers (chopped), 3-4
Lemon juice, 4 tablespoons
Olive oil, 4 tablespoons
Red onion (diced), ½ cup
Salt and pepper to taste
Tomatoes (cored, seeded and chopped), approx 1 pound

Directions

1. In a large bowl, toss in the cucumbers, tomatoes and red onions.

2. Take another bowl and mix olive oil with lemon juice. Add seasonings (salt and pepper) according to your preference.

3. Pour on the tomatoes mixtures and enjoy when chilled.

Chicken Strips
Serves 8-10

Cooking Time

40-50 minutes

Ingredients

Almond flour, 1 cup
Cajun seasoning
Chicken strips (skinless and boneless), 2 lbs
Coconut flour, 3 tablespoons
Coconut milk, 1/8 cup
Eggs, 2
Olive oil
Salt and pepper to taste

Directions

1. Take a bowl and beat in the eggs and the coconut milk.

2. Place the chicken in a glass dish and season with Cajun seasoning, salt and pepper.

3. Top up the chicken with the egg and coconut milk mixture. Let it soak for about 15-20 minutes.

4. In a plate, combine the coconut and almond flour.

5. In a large skillet, heat up the olive oil and taking out one strip at a time, dip it into the flour mixture to coat both sides and place in the skillet.

6. Cook the chicken until it's crispy and thoroughly cooked.

7. Place on a plate and serve.

Paleo Bacon Salad
Serves 3-4

Cooking Time

10 minutes

Ingredients

Asparagus (steamed), 2 bunches
Bacon (cooked and chopped into pieces), 2 cups
Eggs (hard boiled), 2
Champagne vinegar, 1 tablespoon
Dijon mustard, 1 tablespoon
Sea salt, ½ teaspoon
Avocado oil, 3 tablespoons
Coconut oil, 2 tablespoons

Directions

1. Arrange the asparagus on a platter.

2. Take a bowl and mix in salt, vinegar, mustard, avocado oil and coconut oil.

3. Top up the mixture with crumbled eggs and bacon.

4. Enjoy fresh!

Paleo Egg Salad
Serves 8-10

Cooking Time

20 minutes

Ingredients

Uncured bacon, 4 strips

Avocado, 1 large

Hard boiled eggs, 4

Baby spinach, 1 cup

Canned coconut milk, 2 tablespoons

Sea salt, to taste

Pepper, to taste

Directions

1. Mix mashed eggs with coconut milk in a mixing bowl.
2. Add the peeled and pitted avocado and mash again.
3. Add spinach and fold the ingredients together, sprinkle sea salt and pepper to taste.
4. You can have your salad with Paleo bread or serve individually.

Instant Coffee Cake
Serves 1

Cooking Time

5minutes

Ingredients

Almond flour, 2 tablespoons
Apple sauce, 1 tablespoon
Cinnamon, 1 pinch
Coconut oil, 1 tablespoon
Coconut flour, 1 tablespoon
Coconut sugar, 1 tablespoon
Egg (whisked), 1
Maple Syrup, 1 tablespoon
Salt, 1 pinch
Vanilla, 1 teaspoon

Directions

1. Add all ingredients to a large mug and mix well. Make sure to not have any clumps.

2. Put in the microwave for about 3 minutes.

3. Take a small plate and turn over the mug to enjoy your instant, mini coffee cake.

Paleo Yogurt Parfait
Serves 1

Cooking Time

10 minutes

Ingredients

Cashews (unsalted & soaked in water for 20 min), ¾ cp
Coconut meat, 1 cup
Coconut water, 1 cup
Honey for drizzling
Vanilla, 1 teaspoon

Directions

1. Crack the coconut and drain the water into a small bowl.

2. Using a knife cut out the inner meat of the coconut.

3. Add vanilla, coconut meat, coconut water and cashews in a blender. Blend well.

4. Serve with strawberries, blackberries or blueberries as desired and drizzle some honey on the top.

Apple and Coconut Muffins
Serves4

Cooking Time

25 minutes

Ingredients

Almond butter, 1 cup
Almond flour, 1 cup
Apple (cored and chopped), 1
Baking powder, ½ teaspoon
Baking soda, ½ teaspoon
Cinnamon, 1 pinch
Coconut flakes (unsweetened), 1/3 cup
Eggs, 2
Honey, ½ cup
Salt, ¼ teaspoon

Directions

1. Preheat the oven to 350° F.

2. Take a bowl and mix all the ingredients.

3. Grease muffins pan and fill each about ¾ full with the mixture.

4. Bake for 15-20 minutes.

Paleo Meatloaf
Serves 2

Cooking Time

2 hours

Ingredients

Almond meal, 1 can
Egg (raw), 1
Garlic Powder, 1 teaspoon or 2 minced cloves
Ground meat/ground round (completely thawed), 1 pound
Honey, 1/3 or ¼ can (as desired)
Lemon juice, 1 teaspoon
Red bell pepper, ½ large
Tomato paste, 1 6oz can
Tomato puree, ¼ can
White distilled vinegar, ¼ can
Yellow onion, 1 medium

Directions

1.Preheat oven to 375° F.

2. Mix all the ingredients and place in a glass dish.

3. Place in the oven for an hour.

4. Cover the top with a piece of foil and let it set for an additional hour.

5. Your Paleo meatloaf is ready to be served.

Paleo Pancakes
Serves 6-8

Cooking Time

15- 20 minutes

Ingredients

Almond flour (balanced), 1 ½ can
Baking soda, ¼ teaspoon
Celtic sea salt, ¼ teaspoon
Coconut oil, for cooking
Eggs (fresh from pasteurized raised chickens), 3 large
Honey, 2 teaspoons
Vanilla extract, 1 teaspoon
Water, 1 teaspoon

Directions

1. Take a bowl and whisk in the eggs, honey, water and vanilla extract.

2. Add salt, baking soda and almond flour. Stir into a paste of desired consistency.

3. Make pancakes of not more than 3" in diameter and cook on medium low heat.

4. When bubbles form turn and add oil as needed.

5. Serve when golden brown.

Paleo Sweet Tea
Serves 4

Cooking Time

10 minutes

Ingredients

Honey, ½ cup
Ice, 1-2 cubes
Lemon or mint
Tea bags, 2 (family-sized)
Water, 1 quart

Directions

1. Bring the water to boil.

2. Remove from heat and add in the tea bags. Allow it to steep for 5 minutes.

3. Stir in the honey.

4. Take a 2 quart pitcher and pour in the tea.

5. Stir in 1 quart of water.

6. Squeeze in a lemon or add mint as per your preference.

7. Add some ice and enjoy!

Paleo Biscuits and Gravy
Serves 3-4

Cooking Time

60 minutes

Ingredients

For Gravy:

Arrowroot powder, 2 tablespoons
Cayenne pepper, ¼ teaspoon
Country style pork sausage, 16 oz.
Coconut milk, 1 can
Fennel seeds, ¼ teaspoon
Pepper, ½ teaspoon
Sage (dried and rubbed), 1 teaspoon
Salt, ¼ teaspoon

For Biscuits:

Almond flour, ¼ cup
Baking powder, 1 teaspoon
Coconut oil, 1 teaspoon
Coconut flour, ½ cup
Egg whites, 6
Grass-fed butter (cold), 1 tablespoon
Salt, ½ teaspoon

Directions

For Gravy:

1. Take a skillet and heat it over medium-high flame. Brown the sausage cut into small pieces. Set aside.

2. Drain away all the fat, leaving only about a tablespoon behind.

3. Over medium heat, stir in the arrowroot and whisk constantly. Add about 1/3 of the coconut milk slowly while whisking.

4. Mix in the sage, salt, cayenne and salt and pepper.

5. Add back the sausages and cook for a while.

4. Pour over biscuits immediately and serve.

For Biscuits:

1. Preheat oven to 400 F.

2. Take 6 muffin cups and grease with coconut oil.

3. In a food processor, process salt, baking powder, almond flour and coconut flour.

4. Add in the fennel seeds and butter, then process again.

5. Blend in the egg whites until frothy and add them to the food processor. Process.

6. Place the batter into the muffin cups in even quantities filling about ¾ of each.

7. Bake for about 15 minutes or until brown.

8. Enjoy with the gravy!

Almond Flour Paleo Biscuits
Serves 3

Cooking Time

30 minutes

Ingredients

Almond flour (balanced), 3 cups
Baking Soda, ½ teaspoon
Coconut oil (melted), ¼ cup
Eggs, 2
Honey, 1 tablespoon (optional)
Salt, 1 teaspoon

Directions

1. Preheat the oven to 350° F.

2. Take a baking sheet and line it with parchment paper.

3. Take a bowl and add in the salt, baking soda and almond flour.

4. Take another small bowl and whisk in the oil, eggs and honey.

5. Combine both mixtures to form a nice dough.

6. Roll out the dough in a 1-inch thick layer and cut out biscuits using a biscuit cutter.

7. Bake the biscuits for about 12-15 minutes or until golden brown,

Paleo Cat Fish
Serves 2-3

Cooking Time

45 minutes

Ingredients

Almond flour, 2 cups
Catfish fillets, 6
Coconut milk, 1 cup
Egg, 1
Garlic powder, ½ teaspoon
Onion (minced), 1 teaspoon
Paprika, ½ teaspoon
Pepper, 1 teaspoon
Salt, 1 teaspoon
Walnut oil or coconut oil, 1 cup

Directions

1. In a skillet, heat the oil over medium to high flame.

2. Take 1 small and 1 large mixing bowl. In the small bowl, whisk in the coconut milk and egg to form a batter. In the medium bowl, mix the seasonings with the almond flour.

3. Take one skillet at a time. First dip it into the batter and then, shaking off the excess liquid, dip it into the dry mix to coat both sides.

4. Add to the skillet and cook each side for 4-5 minutes. Make sure to turn gently.

5. When golden brown, remove from skillet and put it on a stack of towel papers.

6. Serve immediately or refrigerate for later use.

Paleo Mac n Cheese
Serves 3

Cooking Time

45 minutes

Ingredients

Noodles, 1 pack
Almonds, 4-5
Arrowroot Powder, 4 tablespoons
Coconut oil, 4 tablespoons
Dijon mustard, ½ teaspoon
Coconut milk, 2 ½ cups
Garlic powder, ½ teaspoon
Gluten-free nutritional yeast, 2 heaping tablespoon
Nutmeg, ¼ teaspoon
Onion powder, ½ teaspoon
Paprika (for the orange color), ½ teaspoon
Apple cider Vinegar, 2 tablespoon
Sea salt, 1 teaspoon
Tahini, 1 heaping tablespoon
White wine, 3 tablespoons

Directions

1. Cook the noodles.

2. Take a medium saucepan and heat the coconut oil.

3. Add arrowroot and whisk for 20 seconds.

4. Add coconut milk slowly and whisk into a paste.

5. Bring to boil on low heat.

6. Add in the yeast, mustard, tahini, vinegar, salt, powders, wine, nutmeg and paprika and whisk well.

7. Remove from heat and put it on the side.

8. In a 9 inch casserole pan, place the cooked noodles and the mixture. Blend lightly

9. Sprinkle the almonds and some basil over it.

10. Bake for about 10-12 minutes on 350 F.

Southern Collard Greens and Andouille Sausage
Serves 4

Cooking Time

1 hour 15 minutes

Ingredients

Andouille sausages (paleo-friendly), 4
Apple cider vinegar, 1/3 cup
Bacon (nitrate-free, diced in ¼ inch each), 4-6 slices
Black pepper (freshly grounded), ½ teaspoon
Chicken stock, 1 ¼ cup
Collard greens (rinsed), 2 bunches
Hot Sauce (Frank's original), 1 teaspoon
Onion (diced), 1 cup
Red pepper (crushed), ¼ teaspoon (optional)
Water, ½ cup

Directions

1. Take the collard greens and remove their tough stems. Stack several leaves and cut them crosswise into 2-inch ribbons. Repeat as necessary.

2. Heat a large stockpot or deep skillet over medium-high flame. Sauté bacon for 5-10 minutes or until crispy. Place on paper towel and set aside.

3. Drain all the fat from the skillet, leaving only about 2 tablespoons behind. Sauté onions for 5 minutes.

4. Stir in black pepper, red pepper and collards. Sauté over medium heat for 10 minutes, stirring every 2-3 minutes.

5. Stir in water and 1 cup chicken stock. Cover and simmer for 30-45 minutes.

6. When the liquid has boiled down, stir in the remaining chicken stock and keep the flame high.

7. Stir in hot sauce and vinegar. Cook for 1-2 minutes.

8. Meanwhile follow the package instructions and prepare the sausages. Cut them into slices.

9. Pour in the mixture into a bowl or individual plates. Sprinkle bacon.

10. Serve with sausage slices.

Sweet Potato Pie
Serves 6

Cooking Time

2 hours

Ingredients

For Crust:
Almond flour, 2 ½ cups
Egg (whisked), 1 large
Coconut oil, 2 tablespoon
Sea salt, ½ teaspoon

For Filling:
Sweet potatoes, 1 pound
Coconut oil or ghee (softened), ½ cup
Raw honey, ½ cup
Almond milk, ½ cup
Eggs, 2 large
Ground nutmeg, ¾ teaspoon
Ground cinnamon, ¾ teaspoon
Sea salt, ½ teaspoon
Ginger, ¼ teaspoon
Cardamom, ¼ teaspoon
Vanilla extract, 2 teaspoons

Directions

For Crust:

1. Preheat the oven to 350°F.

2. In a food processor, combine salt and almond flour. Add coconut oil and egg and pulsed into a dough.

3. Wrap the dough into some plastic wrap and refrigerate for about 30 minutes.

4. Press the dough in a pie plate and cover the side up, molding it using your hands.

5. Use a fork to pierce the crust a few times to prevent bubbling during baking

6. Bake for 15 minutes.

7. Let it cool for 10-15 minutes prior to adding the filling.

For Filling:

1. Preheat the oven at 425°F. Bake sweet potato for 40-50 minutes.

2. Let it cool and then, peel off its skin.

3. Take a large bowl and add in the sweet potato and the remaining ingredients.

4. Using a hand mixer, beat the mixture into a smooth paste.

5. Pour on the piecrust.

Bake the pie:

1. Wrap an aluminum foil around the crust edges.

2. Bake the pie for 50-60 minutes at 350°F.

3. Allow cooling before serving.

Tip: Serve with coconut whipped cream.

Paleo Barbecue Sauce Slow-cooker Beef Brisket
Serves 4

Cooking Time

4-6 hours

Ingredients

Beef brisket, 3 lb.
Beef stock (no sugar), 2 cups
Garlic (minced), 3 cloves
Salt and pepper to taste
Sweet onions (sliced), 2

Directions

1. Take a heavy duty freezer bag. Place all the ingredients in it and seal it while making sure all the air is out.

2. The night before serving, place the bag in the fridge and allow defrosting.

3. Using a hot skillet, sear the outside of the meat for 1-2 minutes per side (make sure to not cook it though).

4. Place in a Crockpot and leave on low heat for 6 hours. If you are in a hurry, 4 hours on high heat would do as well.

Fried Okra
Serves 3-4

Cooking Time

35-40 minutes

Ingredients

Flaxseed meal, 1 ½ cups
Frozen Okra, 16 oz (1 bag)
Olive oil, 1 tablespoon
Spices (as per your choice)

Directions

1. Thaw the okra.

2. Toss in remaining ingredients and mix well.

3. Pour in on a baking pan.

4. Bake for 20 minutes at 350 F.

Chicken Salad
Serves4

Cooking Time

25 minutes

Ingredients

Avocados (ripe), 2
Chicken breasts (large), 3
Cilantro (coarsely chopped), 4 tablespoons
Cumin, 1 teaspoon
Dijon mustard, 1 tablespoon
Jalapeno (diced and seeds scrapped out), 1
Lime (juiced), 1
Mayonnaise (Paleo-friendly), 1/3 cup
Poaching liquid (carrots, celery, water, onion, thyme, chicken stock, peppercorns, bay leaf)
Red onion (diced), ¼
Salt and pepper to taste

Directions

1. Take the chicken and season in with salt and pepper.

2. Poach the chicken by placing it in a medium pot, immersing it completely and bring it to boil. Put on low heat, cover in partially and simmer it for 10 minutes. Remove from heat and set aside for 15 minutes before removing the chicken.

3. Allow the chicken to cool down before shredding it with a fork.

4. Add lime juice, mayo, cumin, Dijon, salt and pepper to the chicken. Stir in the cilantro, jalapeno and red onions.

5. Place in the fridge for a few hours.

6. Serve with an avocado and enjoy.

Banana Pudding
Serves 6

Cooking Time

25 minutes

Ingredients

Bananas (very ripe), 3
Cinnamon, ½ teaspoon
Coconut butter, 1 tablespoon
Coconut milk, 1 can
Coconut oil, 1 tablespoon
Egg yolks, 2
Vanilla extract, 1 teaspoon

Directions

5. Turn heat to medium and whisk coconut milk, egg yolks, and vanilla together. Constantly keep stirring until mixture starts to thicken.
6. Remove the mixture from heat and place a small frying pan over medium heat. Heat coconut oil and coconut butter and add slightly mashed bananas with cinnamon. Cook just until bananas start to caramelize.
7. Process the coconut milk and egg mixture in a food processor until it is smooth and creamy.
8. Empty the content in a bowl and refrigerate.
9. Serve chilled.

Fudge
Serves 4

Cooking Time

3-4 hours

Ingredients

Cashews (soaked for 15 min), 1 dl
Coconut Oil, 3 tablespoons
Honey, 2-3 tablespoons
Pecan nut butter, 1 dl
Salt, ½ teaspoon
Vanilla powder, ½ teaspoon

Directions

1. In a food processor, add the cashews and process into a dense butter.

2. Add salt and blend.

3. Add honey, pecan nut butter, coconut oil and vanilla. Process thoroughly.

4. Pour into a 2-3 cm thick rectangle.

5. Cover and refrigerate for at least 3 hours or overnight.

6. Cut into squares.

7. Serve when cold.

Paleo Lemon Bars
Serves

Cooking Time

40 minutes

Ingredients

For the Crust:

Almond flour, 1/2 cup
Coconut oil, 2 1/2 tablespoons
Honey, 2 tablespoons
Unsweetened coconut(shredded), 1 cup
Salt, a pinch
Egg white, 1

For the Filling:

Almond flour, 1/3 cup
Eggs, 3 + 2 egg yolks
Lemon juice, 1/3 cup
Honey, 1/3 cup
Lemon zest, 1 tablespoon (about 2 lemons)

Directions

1. Line a loaf pan with parchment paper and preheat oven to 350 F degrees.
2. Melt coconut oil over medium heat, and add honey, almond flour, shredded coconut, salt and mix well.
3. Add egg white after removing from heat and stir.
4. Bake the mixture for ten minutes.
5. Beat eggs in a large bowl until frothy for the filling. Add the remaining ingredients and beat for 2 minutes more.
6. Pour the filling over the baked crust and bake for 25 minutes.
7. Before serving, let the bars cool. Cut into squares and top with coconut flour or powdered sugar.
8. Store in the fridge in an airtight container for 4 days.

Strawberry Meringues
Serves 5

Cooking Time

3 hours

Ingredients

Arrowroot, ½ teaspoon
Egg whites, 3
Raw honey, 2 tablespoons and 1 teaspoon
Strawberries (sliced), 1 cup
Vanilla, ½ teaspoon

Directions

1. Preheat the oven to 392 F.

2. Take a baking sheet and line it up with parchment paper.

3. Heat a saucepan over medium flame. Stir in the strawberries and 1 tablespoon of honey.

4. Mash the strawberries when they soften up after heating. Remove from heat and pour into a blender or processor. Blend well and place in the refrigerator to cool.

5. Take a bowl and add in the vanilla, egg whites and arrowroot. Whisk well and while continuing to do so, pour in the remaining honey. Whisk until stiff peaks are formed.

6. Whisk in the cooled strawberry mix to form stiff peaks again.

7. Put the mixture in a piping tube and pipe it onto the parchment paper into mounds

8. Bake for 2.5 hours and remove from oven. In the last 30 minutes, turn off the heat.

9. Store in an airtight container after meringues have completely cooled and enjoy!

Apple Fritters
Serves 4

Cooking Time

15 minutes

Ingredients

Apples (Granny Smith), 4
Cinnamon, 1 teaspoon
Coconut (shredded), ¼ cup
Coconut Flour, 1 tablespoon
Coconut oil
Eggs, 5
Flaxmeal, ¼ cup
Honey, 2 tablespoon (optional)
Nutmeg, 1/8 teaspoon
Salt, ¼ teaspoon

Directions

1. Use a hand grater to shred the apples and pat with paper towels.

2. Mix with the remaining ingredients.

3. Take a heavy-bottomed skillet and heat the coconut oil over medium-high flame.

4. Fry spoonfuls of the batter poured into the skillet, frying each side for 2-3 minutes each.

5. Pour on to paper towels to drain off excess oil.

6. Serve hot with almond butter or honey.

Cashew Cheesecake
Serves 8

Cooking Time

25-30 minutes

Ingredients

For the Crust:

Coconut (raw and flaked), ¼ cup
Dates (soft pitted), ½ cup
Raw Pecans, ½ cup
Sea salt, 1 pinch

For the Filling:

Agave nectar, 2/3 cup
Cashews (raw, soaked and drained), 3 ½ cups
Extra virgin olive oil, 2/3 cup
Lemon juice (fresh), 2/3 cup
Vanilla extract, 2 teaspoons

Directions

1. Soak the nuts and set aside.

2. Chop the nuts, coconut, dates and salt into the food processor bowl. Process it to make the crust and set aside.

3. Warm the coconut oil in a bowl of warm water.

4. Pour in the coconut oil, lemon juice, agave, vanilla and cashews into the pitcher of a blender. Blend well until completely smooth.

5. Take an8 inch pan and smooth the crust into it. Give proper attention to the sides.

6. Top it up with the filling and freeze for at least 4 hours or overnight.

7. Before serving, let it thaw for about 30 minutes and cut into small pieces.

Coconut Lemon Meltaways
Serves 8-10

Cooking Time

20-25 minutes

Ingredients

Almond flour, 1 ½ cup
Coconut (dried, shredded and unsweetened), 1 ½ cups
Coconut flour, 1/3 cup
Coconut oil, ¼ cup and 1 tablespoon (divided)
Lemon juice, 4 tablespoons
Lemon zest, 1 tablespoon
Maple Syrup or Raw organic honey, 6 tablespoons
Salt, 2 pinches (big ones)
Vanilla, 2 teaspoons

Directions

1. Take a bowl and mix in the almond flour, coconut, coconut flour and salt. Set aside.

2. Use a small mixing bowl and pour in lemon juice, lemon zest, vanilla and maple syrup. Combine well with the dry ingredients by slowly streaming in the mixture with an electric mixer.

3. Stream in the coconut oil while mixing. As the oil starts cooling, it would thicken the mixture.

4. Form small round cookies of the mixtures and arrange on a sheet.

5. Serve immediately by either warming them for an hour or more, or by keeping them in the fridge. Doing one of the two is essential to prevent the texture of the cookies to be soft and moist.

Chocolate Chip Cookies
Serves 10-15

Cooking Time

20-25 minutes

Ingredients

Almond flour (balanced), 3 cups
Baking soda, ¾ teaspoon
Coconut flour (organic), 1 tablespoon
Eggs (large), 2
Enjoy Life, 1 package
Kosher salt, 1 ¼ teaspoons
Molasses (unsulphured), 1 ½ teaspoons
Organic blonde coconut palm sugar, ¼ cup
Organic ghee (melted), ¼ cup
Organic light wave nectar, ½ cup
Organic palm shortening, ¼ cup
Pure vanilla extract, 1 ½ tablespoons
Semi-sweet Chocolate Mega Chunks (chopped)

Directions

1. Take a large mixing bowl and add in the salt, baking soda and the flours. Whisk together and set aside.

2. In a food processor, combine ghee, shortening and sugar. Process for a minute.

3. Add in the remaining ingredients and process into a smooth and creamy paste.

4. Combine the flour mixture to form a completely blended and smooth dough.

5. Add chocolate chips and let it rest (uncovered) for 15 minutes at room temperature.

6. Place two oven racks in the middle of the oven and preheat it to 350°F.

7. Take two insulated baking sheet and line each with parchment paper. Set aside.

Orange and Almond Cake
Serves 5

Cooking Time

15 minutes

Ingredients

Almond meal (blanched), 2 ½ cups
Baking powder, 1 teaspoon
Eggs, 6
Natvia, 50g
Navel Oranges, 2
Xylitol, 100g

Directions

1. Wash the unpeeled oranges.

2. Boil in a pot for 2 hours. Change water after an hour.

3. Drain water and set aside to cool.

4. Preheat the oven to 356 F.

5. Take a blender or a mixing bowl, break in the eggs and stir in the Natvia and Xylitol. Blend well.

6. Process the chopped and unpeeled oranges in a food processor to form a smooth mixture.

7. Blend the orange mixture into the egg mixture.

8. Add the baking powder and the almond meal. Mix.

9. Cover a baking pan with a 20 cm baking paper.

10. Bake batter in the baking pan for 1 hour or until its top turns golden brown.

Bon-Bons
Serves 3-4

Cooking Time

15 minutes

Ingredients

Almond butter, ½ cup
Coconut sugar, ¼ cup
Dark Chocolate, 2 cups
Dates (chopped), ½ cup
Ground Almonds, ½ cup

Directions

1. Take a bowl and add in walnuts, almond butter, dates and the sugar. Mix well.

2. Make ½ inch balls of the mixture and arrange on a plate.

3. Using a double broiler, melt the chocolate.

4. Coat each ball properly with the chocolate.

5. Place on wax paper and allow it to cool.

6. Put in the freezer or the fridge.

7. Enjoy!

Sweet Potato Brownies
Serves 4-6

Cooking Time

50 minutes

Ingredients

Baking powder, ¼ teaspoon
Cinnamon, ¼ teaspoon
Cocoa powder (unsweetened), 2 tablespoons
Coconut flour, 3 tablespoons
Coconut oil, ¼ cup
Dark chocolate chips, ½ cup
Eggs (whisked), 3
Raw honey, 1/3 cup
Salt, 1 pinch
Sweet Potatoes (small to medium), 2
Vanilla extract, ½ teaspoon

Directions

1. Boil the sweet potatoes until soft. Take a bowl, remove skin and mash the potatoes.

2. Preheat the oven to 350° F.

3. First add all your wet ingredients to the sweet potatoes and then, add in all the dry ingredients.

4. Mix for 1-2 minutes on a low to medium flame.

5. Add the mixture to an 8x8 glass and bake for 30-35 minutes.

6. Allow to cool before serving.

Snicker Doodles
Serves 4

Cooking Time

25 minutes

Ingredients

Almond butter, ½ cup
Almond flour, 2 cups
Baking soda, 1 teaspoon
Cinnamon, 2 teaspoons and 1 tablespoon (divided)
Eggs, 2
Natural honey, 1 tablespoon
Maple Syrup, ½ cup
Palm shortening, ½ cup
Vanilla, 2 tablespoons

Directions

1. Add the almond butter, eggs, palm shortening, maple syrup and vanilla into a bowl. Beat until smooth.

2. Take a bowl and mix in flour, soda and 2 teaspoons of cinnamon.

3. Add the dry mixture to the wet mixture. Blend well.

4. Make cookies on a greased cookie sheet using a tablespoon to pour in the mixture and spread it into a flat cookie. Remember to leave space between the cookies and keep the cookies about ½ inches thick.

5. Combine sugar and cinnamon (1 tablespoon) in a separate bowl and sprinkle over the cookies, ideally 1/8 of the combination for each cookie.

6. Bake for 8-10 minutes or until golden brown on 350° F.

&. Allow to cool for an hour at least before you serve or store them in airtight jars.

Strawberry Pie
Serves 4

Cooking Time

60 minutes

Ingredients

For Paleo Pie Crust:

Almond flour, 2 cups
Egg whites, 3 tablespoons or egg yolk, 1
Ghee or unsalted butter, ¼ cup
Salt, 1 pinch

For Strawberry Filling:

Arrowroot powder, 1/3 cup
Coconut sugar, 1/3 cup
Lemon juice, 2 tablespoons
Strawberries (quartered), 4 ½ cups

Directions

1. Preheat the oven to 400° F.

2. Put all the ingredients of the pie crust in a bowl and whip them into a consistent paste.

3. Pour into a greased pan. Turn the oven to 350° F and bake for 15 minutes.

4. Take another bowl and add in all the ingredients of the strawberry filling. Mix well.

5. Add to the pre-baked pie. Bake for an additional 25 minutes.

6. Set the oven temperature at 375 °F and bake for 10 minutes.

7. Remove from oven and allow it to cool before you serve.

Roasted Beef Spinach Salad
Serves 4

Cooking Time

10 minutes

Ingredients

Apple (Granny Smith), 1 (cut in chunks)
Bacon slices, 2-3
Beets, 3-4
Horseradish, 2 teaspoon
Maple syrup, 1 tablespoon
Olive oil, 3 tablespoon
Parmesan cheese (shavings), (optional)
Red wine vinegar, 2 tablespoons
Salt and pepper, ¼ teaspoon each
Spinach

Directions

1. Scrub the beets and remove their tops, cutting them off about one inch from the bulb.

2. Wrap up each beet separately in foil.

3. Using a baking sheet, roast the beets on 425° F for about 60 minutes.

4. Allow to cool and cut into chunks.

5. Cook the bacon until it's crispy.

6. In a bowl, whisk together horseradish, maple syrup, olive oil, parmesan cheese, red wine vinegar, and salt and pepper.

7. Place spinach in a bowl and toss in the bacon, beets, apple and dressing. Toss well.

Cucumber, Tomato and Onion Salad
Serves 4-6

Cooking Time

15 minutes

Ingredients

Cucumbers (Peeled and thinly sliced), 2
Cherry tomatoes (halved), 1 pint
Onion (thinly sliced), ½
Fresh Parsley leaves (chopped), 2 tablespoons
Apple Cider Vinegar, 1 tablespoon
Olive oil, 1 tablespoon
Salt and pepper (freshly grounded) to taste

Directions

1. Toss in all ingredients in a large serving bowl. Mix well.

2. Allow to set for 10 minutes.

3. Serve.

Conclusion

Adopting a Paleo diet is a great way to eating healthy and staying healthy. Now that you have an array of recipes at your disposal, time to transform your diet plan and try out new, delicious recipes that can address health concerns and provide you essential nutrition.